Chronic Fatigue Syndrome

Everything You Need to Know About Chronic Fatigue Syndrome, Treatments, and Diet Plans to Lead a Productive Life

By Cailin Chase

Disclaimers

The information in this book is not intended as medical advice or a substitute for consultation with your healthcare provider. This information should be used in conjunction with the advice of your own healthcare practitioner. Always consult with your physician prior to changing and/or discontinuing medications or diet.

Any trademarks or product names used in this publication are the property of their owners, and are for identification only, and no claim implied by their use.

Chronic Fatigue Syndrome

Table of Contents

Introduction

Although the medical sciences have come a long way in the last century or so, there are still many conditions which remain largely misunderstood. One such condition is Chronic Fatigue Syndrome, also known as myalgic encephalomyelitis.

Chronic fatigue syndrome is an umbrella term for a collection of unpleasant symptoms, chiefly tiredness and fatigue as the name would suggest. Owing the lack of full understanding of the condition, conventional medicine and its practitioners find it difficult to even know where to start when it comes to helping you, their patient.

This book aims to help you gain a better understanding of just what chronic fatigue syndrome is and how you can minimise its debilitating symptoms and regain control of your life. We'll take a look at its symptoms and the process of diagnosis, which is unfortunately a diagnosis of exclusion due to the lack of concrete medical knowledge of the causes and treatment.

We'll discuss the conventional methods for attempting to combat chronic fatigue particularly based upon the idea that adrenal fatigue, the wearing out of your body's natural stress response system. Though even conventional medicine recognises the need for a more holistic approach than usual for the treatment of chronic fatigue syndrome, it advocates cognitive behavioural therapy and dietary change but little else.

As we are not merely physical beings, this book aims to explore the holistic therapies purported to help deal with the symptoms and effects of chronic fatigue syndrome on you as a whole person and not just a purely physical organism. These holistic therapies vary in approach and originate from different parts of the globe, involving different concepts of diseases and subsequently methods of treatment.

It has been long recognised that diet has a significant effect on our overall health and well-being, and as such this book will conclude with some dietary advice and some recipes to help you to put this advice into practice and overcome your fatigue.

What is Chronic Fatigue Syndrome?

Chronic fatigue syndrome, as its name would suggest, is characterised primarily by fatigue that does not diminish after what would usually be considered adequate rest. Its cause is unknown and there are a multitude of symptoms which unfortunately overlap with many common diseases. This is what makes it difficult for your doctor to quickly diagnosis your exact condition.

It is generally recognised that the following symptoms constitute what is referred to as chronic fatigue syndrome:

- Fatigue without obvious cause that does not diminish upon rest
- Insomnia and ineffective sleep
- Muscle and joint pain
- Headaches
- Painful lymph nodes (for example, in the armpits or in the neck)
- Sore throat
- Difficulty with mental tasks
- Flu-like symptoms
- Dizziness
- Nausea
- Heart palpitations
- Digestive complaints (constipation, in particular)

These symptoms tend to worsen after any kind of exertion, including mental, and fatigue can last up to a whole day after the activity in question. The symptoms are wide-ranging and really not very specific and a number of different diseases are suspected before chronic fatigue syndrome. It is of course very frustrating to have your symptoms disregarded or overlooked, but conventional medicine takes the approach that other more common, better understood diseases should be ruled out before a diagnosis of chronic fatigue syndrome is made.

Typically, the kinds of diseases first suspected by your doctor are likely to be those commonly associated with fatigue as the main symptom. Naturally, this includes sleep disorders such as obstructive sleep apnea which can be tested for and thus ruled out quite quickly.

A simple blood test can rule out a number of medical conditions such as anaemia and low thyroid activity, which commonly affect women more than men. Also, a blood sugar test can rule out diabetes, which often leaves people feeling constantly tired without having exerted themselves particularly.

Increasingly, conventional medical practitioners are recognising the importance of mental health alongside physical and as such a number of psychological conditions have been associated with chronic fatigue. It would be wise to speak to a qualified practitioner to rule out such issues as depression and bipolar disorder, which can contribute significantly to a feeling of tiredness and fatigue.

Only once these kinds of conditions have been eliminated will most doctors think about a diagnosis of chronic fatigue syndrome. They are most often reluctant to make such a diagnosis due to the fact that it is a largely misunderstood condition and not something that is easily fixed, unlike some of the other potential diagnoses.

This is not to say that chronic fatigue syndrome cannot be overcome. Understanding some of the potential causes of chronic fatigue syndrome can help us to work out how to minimise the symptoms and gain some control over our life and everyday activities.

There is a wide range of potential causes of chronic fatigue syndrome but unfortunately there doesn't seem to be a common denominator between each of them. It may be that chronic fatigue syndrome is the result of a number of different causes acting in one or more ways. Potential causes include:

- Nutritional deficiencies (including vitamin D and magnesium)
- Acute stress (physical and/or psychological)
- Infections (such as Epstein-Barr virus)
- Digestive health issues (gut dysfunction or gut flora imbalance)

The nutritional causes will be discussed further in the dietary advice included later on in this book as it has been considered of more use to present each potential deficiency followed immediately by advice with which to combat it.

One of the most recent bodily mechanisms purported to have a major role in the development of chronic fatigue syndrome is the stress management system known as the hypothalamus-pituitary-adrenal axis. This involves two separate parts of the brain and part of the glands which are found just above each kidney. This is a natural feedback loop system which works by each component in the loop responding to a high concentration of compounds formed lower down in the axis by shutting down production. To put it simply, the body regulates the production of stress hormones by shutting down production when too much has been made.

It is thought that chronic fatigue syndrome may at least in part be a result of a constant stressor acting upon the body. The long term presence of any stressor causes the adrenal glands to produce high levels of adrenaline and cortisol, the hormones involved in short term and long term response to stress respectively. Over time, the adrenal glands become exhausted and overused such that they are no longer able to mount a proper response to stress. This adrenal fatigue leaves your whole body and as a result you as a whole person tired and unable to function as you would wish.

The normal function of cortisol in its role as a long term responder to stress is to promote the function of the immune system. Too little cortisol, as is often the case in chronic fatigue syndrome following adrenal fatigue, and the body becomes susceptible to infections and autoimmune diseases.

The problematic thing with the link between the adrenal glands and chronic fatigue syndrome is that the stress that contributes to this fatigue and while these glands are the body's natural defence against stress they are also the first tissues in your body to shut down in the face of chronic, unrelenting stressors.

Adrenal fatigue and subsequently chronic fatigue syndrome are becoming increasingly common as a result of the changes in modern lifestyle such as increased caffeine intake, poor sleep patterns and poor diet.

Whatever the cause or combination thereof, there are many things offered by conventional medicine as well as by holistic therapies to improve the symptoms of chronic fatigue syndrome. It is believed that the best approach to this condition is to adopt an approach that considers you as a whole person, including both physical and psychological factors, in order to treat your specific condition. You may find a range of approaches beneficial and these will be discussed in the next chapter.

Conventional Treatment

The typical approach of conventional medical practitioners is to recommend some lifestyle changes in order to adapt to the constraints of your condition. Also, cognitive behavioural therapy has been extensively investigated as a suitable means of minimising the effects of symptoms through the development of effective coping mechanisms.

Generally speaking, the approach of conventional medicine towards chronic fatigue syndrome once it has finally been diagnosed is reasonably holistic. The aim is to increase your physical capabilities while simultaneously working on your emotional and psychological outlook on your condition.

Your doctor is likely to recommend that you attend a **graded exercise course** with an accredited physiotherapist. The purpose of such a course is to start with gentle exercises aimed at improving your range of motion and slowly build up over time to more strenuous yet manageable exercises. This is aimed at allowing you to gradually develop muscle strength and endurance, this minimising the effects of chronic fatigue syndrome.

To start with a trained specialist will look at you as an individual and recommend some simple forms of exercise that you can do in order to improve the physical side of your symptoms. This usually involves swimming or walking to raise your heart rate slightly. This kind of gentle approach allows you to develop your strength and endurance in a manageable way that means that you can feel the positive effects of gradually building up your abilities.

Another physical approach to chronic fatigue syndrome is the **management of your activity** in general. You'll be asked to complete an activity diary which will show your doctor the kinds of activities you are able to complete and the lengths of time you are able to spend on doing these activities. Your doctor can then advise you about different ways in which you can slowly increase different aspects of each activity, thus further developing your stamina.

As an adjunct to this physical approach, many doctors now recommend that you undertake some **cognitive behavioural therapy**. This is a form of client-centred psychological counselling that promotes ideas of how to understand and cope wit your condition and thus alter your behaviour to better influence your condition. Simply feeling in control of your own situation through this kind of therapy can work wonders on your general well-being and approach to your own life. It is amazing how much a change in outlook can alter the physical side of things for the better.

Cognitive behavioural therapy begins by looking at breaking down big problems into smaller, more manageable parts so that you can focus on the individual components of a problem and build up a solution from the bottom. This approach can help you to come to terms with your diagnosis and challenge any issues you have that may be preventing you from overcoming some of your symptoms.

Incidentally, the use of this kind of therapy does not necessarily mean that chronic fatigue syndrome is a psychological condition. Rather, it is used to help you manage your approach to your symptoms and it has been shown to be successful in this sense for patients with all sorts of diseases.

As you might expect, another approach to chronic fatigue syndrome is the **use of pharmaceutical drugs**. The only issue with this is that it is not like a simple infection which can be easily treated by taking an antibiotic for a week and then forgetting all about it. Being that chronic fatigue syndrome is poorly understood, such medications are taken to relieve symptoms, rather than actually cure or prevent your condition. With that said, there are still some benefits to be reaped from taking certain kinds of medicines.

Over-the-counter pain relieving medications can be used to ease some of the physical symptoms such as muscle and joint aches and pains. Additionally, your doctor may be able to prescribe something a little stronger for those times where your usual medication doesn't cut the mustard. However, the stronger the drug, the stronger the side effects or risks tend to be. As such, these kinds of drugs should not be taken for prolonged period of time. Instead, you might be referred to a specialist pain management clinic where they will know better how to manage your pain, whether it is with more specific medication or a non-physical approach.

Commonly, drugs are prescribed that are usually used for cases of depression. This is not because your doctor thinks that your symptoms are psychological in nature, or that there is no true physical component to your condition, but rather it is because such drugs have been long associated with a positive effect on pain and insomnia. These are two big issues when it comes to chronic fatigue syndrome, and so-called antidepressants such as amitriptyline can be very helpful.

With many chronic conditions, feelings of depression or low mood are naturally a problem. After all, no one wants to have to live long term with such symptoms. This means that you can use such drugs to combat some aspects of the psychological impact that chronic fatigue syndrome has on you as a person, as well as dealing with the pain and sleep problems. This is not to say, however, that such medications are a substitute for further investigation and resolution of any issues you may have with coping with your condition.

Though the advice of a doctor is often indispensable, the lack of understanding associated with chronic fatigue syndrome means that a number of holistic therapies may be useful as an adjunct to the therapy options promoted by conventional medicine. These options will be evaluated in the next chapter.

Holistic Therapies

Diet and Lifestyle Changes

Seeing as how chronic fatigue syndrome affects your life in a global manner, it is easy to see how making a few diet and lifestyle changes may have a significant influence on your condition. With the right changes you'll give yourself a fighting chance and be able to better cope with the effects of your fatigue.

There have been many **nutritional deficiencies** that have been suggested as being causative in chronic fatigue syndrome. Changing your intake of different nutrients is probably the simplest way in which you can make a positive impact on your condition.

There seems to be a correlation between **low vitamin D levels** and chronic fatigue syndrome. It is not clear, however, whether this is a causative factor or if it is just that sufferers of chronic fatigue syndrome tend to be able to go outside less than the average person and as such have less exposure to sunlight.

As vitamin D is produced in the skin following contact with ultraviolet light from the sun, the simplest way to get more access to sunlight without great exertion is to sit out in the garden or similar. Some vitamin D is obtained from the diet, in particular from cold water fish, so it may be possible to increase your intake this way.

It has also been suggested that **magnesium deficiency** has a link to chronic fatigue syndrome. Normally, magnesium is used by the body for literally hundreds of metabolic processes but is particularly vital for nerve and muscle function, being responsible for steadying the heartbeat, allowing muscle tissue to relax and it is also involved in the control of energy production. Even considering just these functions of many, it is obvious how magnesium deficiency may affect the severity of chronic fatigue syndrome even it is is not necessarily a causative factor.

Fortunately, there are many ways in which we can increase our body's intake and use of magnesium to relieve fatigue and control other physical symptoms such as heart palpitations, the conscious awareness and feeling of your heart beating in your chest.

Many of us consume far too many carbonated beverages, that is to say soda drinks, and darker colored drinks such as cola tend to contain phosphates. These chemical compounds are responsible for binding magnesium before it is absorbed by your gut, such that it is unavailable for use by the body. Simply by avoiding the consumption of soda during meals could help to improve your symptoms.

Furthermore, these soda drinks are often full of caffeine which is a diuretic, meaning that it makes you urinate more. This causes the kidneys to excrete magnesium regardless of whether your body has a deficiency of it. As a result, it would be best to avoid all caffeinated beverages including tea and coffee. The same concept applies to alcoholic beverages, so it would be ideal to eliminate such drinks from your diet.

Magnesium levels are also affected by stress levels. As mentioned previously in this book, the body's adrenal system, its stress control system, is often altered for the worse in such conditions as chronic fatigue syndrome. An increase in adrenaline and cortisol, both produced by the adrenal glands, has been associated with lower magnesium levels. Finding a way in which to reduce your stress levels is important for many reasons, but may particularly be related to improving your magnesium levels and thus increasing your energy.

Unfortunately many conventional pharmaceutical medicines have a wide range of untoward side effects on the body, and this includes an effect on magnesium levels. Such drugs include diuretics (water tablets), birth control, hormone replacement therapy and some heart medications. While it is often vital that you take these medications, it might be worthwhile asking your doctor whether some of these drugs are having an effect on your magnesium levels. If so, you could request that any non-essential drugs are removed from your regular prescription. Remember to always ask your physician first before you stop taking any medicines that they have prescribed. This advice is not a substitute for a fully qualified medical doctor who can see you and examine you in person.

Magnesium may also be reduced or poorly absorbed as a result of certain mineral supplements. Though it is often beneficial to consume extra vitamins and minerals in the form of supplements, calcium in particular causes magnesium to be more poorly absorbed by the body. As such, it is very important to take calcium and magnesium supplements in a 1:1 ratio to ensure that the beneficial effects of proper intake of both minerals are obtained. A magnesium chloride supplement may also be useful as the chloride content can be used to improve gut health and digestion.

Alternatively, some magnesium can be found in your diet. Such foods include spinach, avocado, nuts and most forms of meat and fish.

Being that the main symptom you are likely to be experiencing is fatigue, a tiredness that does not go away even with plenty of rest, it make sense that your body may not be producing energy in the manner in which it ought to be. One compound involved in almost all bodily methods of generating energy is known as **coenzyme Q10**. Studies have shown that people suffering from chronic fatigue syndrome have a lower level of this compound in their blood than people who do not have symptoms of fatigue.

Some studies have shown that coenzyme Q10 supplementation can reduce the intensity and frequency of headaches, a common symptom of chronic fatigue syndrome. Fortunately coenzyme Q10 is a substance which can easily be incorporated into your diet in the form of a supplement. It is also prevalent in organ meats such as heart, liver and kidneys so if possible find a way to include these foods in your diet. One such delicious way might be the consumption of pâté made from liver.

A further dietary link between chronic fatigue syndrome and nutritional efficiency is found in the case of vitamin B3, also known as **niacin**. Amongst other functions, niacin is involved in the formation of nicotinamide adenine dinucleotide (NAD). The addition and removal of hydrogen to this compound to make NADH is part of the energy-generating apparatus of every cell of your body. As such, a deficiency in niacin may lead to a feeling of fatigue.

One small study has shown that supplementation with NADH has a positive effect on the symptoms of chronic fatigue syndrome. Though further studies are required to establish this finding, you may get some benefit from taking such a supplement.

The production of energy in the cells of your body involved tiny components known as mitochondria. If these are not working properly or cannot receive the kinds of nutrients they require to function, then the result is that you'll feel tired and sluggish. One compound involved in helping these mitochondria get the fuel they need is known as **L-carnitine**.

Without a sufficient intake of this compound, people often complain of muscle pain, fatigue and a reduced exercise tolerance. With the similarity of such symptoms to chronic fatigue syndrome, it is being increasingly acknowledged that supplementation with L-carnitine may help to reduce the symptoms of your condition by facilitating the production of energy within your body.

The link between chronic fatigue syndrome and certain infections such as those caused by the Epstein-Barr virus has led to the idea that there is some kind of immunological process going on. For example, a link has been documented between type 1 diabetes and chronic fatigue syndrome. This form of diabetes is ultimately genetic and autoimmune in nature and is not the same as type 2 diabetes which is often acquired from a lifetime of poor dietary choices.

What seems to be the case is that those of us who suffer from chronic fatigue syndrome are for some reason unable to mount an immune response to such infectious microorganisms as the Epstein-Barr virus and cytomegalovirus. This failure to completely eradicate the source of disease is thought to lead to a chronic state of disease, and as such many forms of effective treatment are unsurprisingly targeted at boosting the immune system or related bodily processes.

People who suffer with chronic fatigue syndrome frequently complain of pain in their muscles and joints as well as problems with their digestion. The common association between irritable bowel syndrome, muscular pain and chronic fatigue occurs often enough that a causative link between the three conditions is assumed to exist.

As diet is so important to our general health and well-being regardless of such symptoms, it would make a lot of sense to make dietary alterations to support gut health. Such changes include the consumption of **prebiotic and probiotic foods** in order to support the colonisation of your gut by beneficial intestinal bacteria and not those which promote disease states. Such a diet involves a high consumption of fruits and vegetables as well as fermented foods such as yogurt or sauerkraut.

Some studies have been done to investigate the specific dietary changes required in order to reduce the symptoms of chronic fatigue syndrome. Most such studies tend to be small and thus may not apply to everyone who suffers from fatigue, but are nevertheless worth looking in to. One such study involved the adoption of a diet prohibiting things like processed grains and dairy, that is to say it was perhaps the kind of diet that our ancestors would have enjoyed before the advent of agriculture and animal husbandry.

Combined with adequate sleep and rest, a plan to manage stress, plus the consumption of some supplementary vitamins and minerals, the patients involved in this study did in fact report that their symptoms had reduced in severity. A diet such as this would be anti-inflammatory and generally good for the digestive system so it may be worth avoiding grain-based foods and non-fermented dairy products to see if it has any benefit for you as an individual.

Herbal Remedies

Before the advent of modern medicine, our ancestors relied primarily on their knowledge of natural compounds found in the plants around them in order to heal their ailments and provide symptomatic relief. Before the scientific method was developed, there was no way to prove beyond doubt the efficacy of such herbs and it is only now that such studies are being done. As such, the empirical evidence for some herbal remedies is lacking somewhat.

However, this does not mean that you cannot find use for such herbs. After all, many of the most commonly used medications were either directly derived from herbal compounds or their invention was inspired by the chemical action of similar natural chemical substances. One of the most well known of such medications is aspirin, which is found in natural form in willow bark. The bark of this tree was ground to a powder and used by the Ancient Greeks as a pain reliever. It was even mentioned by Hippocrates, often considered the father of modern medicine.

One of the most frequently used herbs to fight the effects of tiredness and fatigue is **ginseng**. This is a herb widely used in Asia and is an integral component of many herbal remedies originating in China. Some studies have shown that ginseng is effective at reducing the fatigue associated with chronic fatigue syndrome.

In particular, Panax ginseng has a positive effect on the mononuclear cells of the immune system. These are the cells affected by the Epstein-Barr virus commonly associated with chronic fatigue syndrome. These cells are crucial in the proper functioning of the immune system and this form of ginseng may have a significant effect on your symptoms.

Traditional Chinese Medicine

One of the major ways in which traditional Chinese medicine has contributed to modern healthcare is to be found in acupuncture. It is a holistic approach which takes into account all aspects of your individual being. Acupuncture makes use of very fine, sterilised needles to affect the body's energy through the skin.

The fundamental energy possessed by all living things is known as "Qi" and it is this vital force that is manipulated by means of acupuncture. It is considered that Qi runs through our bodies along channels known as meridians and that each organ is affected by the balance of this Qi.

Qi is considered to have two opposing yet balancing aspects known as yin and yang. Generally speaking, rest corresponds to "yin" whereas activity corresponds to "yang". This concept is used in acupuncture alongside the concept of there being a five element system in nature.

The five elements of nature are represented by Wood and Fire as being more "yang", Water and Metal being more "yin", and Earth being a balance between the two. Each organ as a functional system is considered to be related to each one of these elements and an acupuncturist will assess overall health according to the effects of yin and yang on a person life force.

A diagnosis is made by means of feeling for a number of pulses on the wrist and tender points on the body, combined with a general enquiry about your health and state of mind. It is difficult to comprehend this approach to treatment for many of us in the West, who are not accustomed to this kind of philosophy let alone this kind of medicine.

That said, with conditions that are as poorly understood as chronic fatigue syndrome, it may well be worth investigating a treatment modality such as acupuncture. It is well known for its ability to relieve stress and this alone may have a positive contribution to make towards your recovery or improvement of symptoms.

In fact, chronic fatigue syndrome is a condition known to traditional Chinese medicine and there are several theories or causative mechanisms to do with it. These are as follows:

- Spleen Qi deficiency
- Kidney yin deficiency
- Essence deficiency
- Kidney yang deficiency

Spleen Qi deficiency is particularly associated with dampness and chronic disease and is something that is commonly addressed by Chinese medicine including acupuncture and dietary change, much of which is similar to dietary advice contained in this book.

Kidney yin deficiency is particularly associated wi dryness and aching bones and joints. It is considered likely that other organ systems are involved in such yin deficiency within the framework of Chinese medicine as the kidneys are considered the root of the body.

In this capacity the essence of the body, or Jing, emanates from the kidneys and determines the body's overall constitution. It is believed to form the basis of growth and development, and a loss of this is implicated in susceptibility to disease. The constant acquisition of infections and allergies is considered to be directly related to a loss of essence through an imbalance in work versus play, and activity versus rest.

Finally, kidney yang deficiency is associated with bodily weakness and slowed metabolism. The importance of the kidney in the traditional Chinese approach to chronic fatigue syndrome cannot be understated, and there are many therapies that have been devised based on this. These include herbal supplements and acupuncture. The latter is particularly useful for stress release and may benefit you in this manner in an additional to any physical restorative properties that it may have.

Ayurveda

Ayurveda, the traditional Indian form of medicine, much like the Chinese medicine discussed earlier in the chapter, focuses on the person as a whole and is based on an understanding of the person's individual constitution. Ayurveda promotes the idea of detoxification through the use of herbs and diet to aid digestion and thus overall health and well-being.

It has been believed throughout history that the gut is the source of all illness, that is to say that if you eat poorly then you will succumb to disease. There is clearly some truth to this, and **there is a definite link between the consumption of a properly balanced diet rich in vitamins and minerals and good health**. From this point of view, Ayurvedic medicine seems to have something to offer sufferers of chronic fatigue syndrome.

Generally speaking, health is considered to be optimal when there is balance between the three bodily humours or principles, also known as dosha.

Vata is the impulse principle and is associated with wind. It is responsible for the correct functioning of the nervous system.

Pitta is the bilious humour and is mostly associated with heat. It is responsible for the correct functioning of the bowels, liver, spleen amongst other organs and as such is considered to be the main driver of digestion and metabolism.

Kapha is the bodily fluid principle and is associated with the carriage of nutrients throughout the body as well as the production of mucus.

The balance of these three components is further influenced by the kind of constitution that your body has according to Ayurvedic principles. This in turn dictates the specific approach that a practitioner would take to treat your condition.

Practitioners of Ayurveda believe that there are four general causes of fatigue:

- Overuse of the body
- Underuse of the body
- Unhealthy diet
- Irregular sleep

Chronic fatigue syndrome is considered ultimately to be a condition of imbalance of vata, the wind impulse associated with nervous function. As such, you would be recommended to consume foods which control vata and help to restore energy. Some advice in this respect might include the introduction of hot soups and foods that are mildly spiced. The spice component of the food is significant in that it should be spiced enough to reap the benefit of the constituent spices without overloading.

Cold foods and drinks, in particular cold water and cream, are discouraged in the treatment of chronic fatigue syndrome as they are considered to aggravate kapha. A low protein diet is also advocated as protein-rich foods such as meat are relatively difficult to digest and produce large quantities of waste substances full of nitrogen. Just as with conventional Western medicine, caffeinated and sugary soda drinks are prohibited as they contribute to further fatigue despite the initial boost they may give to energy.

The specific spices suggested for use in treatment for chronic fatigue syndrome depend on the specific cause identified. Overuse of the body, that is to say activity that oversteps the body's limits, may be treated with foods incorporating black pepper and fenugreek. Additionally, some types of nuts may of use, such as almonds and walnuts.

According to Ayurvedic principles, the second general cause of such fatigue is underuse of the body. The idea is that if the body is not used at the optimal level then it will degenerate and lose its function due to the accumulation of toxic substances, known collectively as "ama". The treatment of such a phenomenon is another way in which the Ayurvedic approach coincides with modern medicine: in the advocation of gentle exercise. In this case, yoga is the preferred method of exercise and provides a gentle and relaxing way to introduce physical activity into your lifestyle. Yoga teachers tend to be very accommodating to each of their students needs and this can be a great way to increase social interaction as well as improve symptoms.

A focus on the importance of food is integral to the Ayurvedic concept of health, and food is considered divine and thus to eat improperly is to disrespect and disregard the vital nature of it. Certain foods are believed to sap the body of energy, leaving you lethargic and contributing towards your symptoms. If is advised that you consume foods which are easily digested so that you can reduce the problems you have of incorrectly nourishing the body, mind and spirit. Such foods include whole grains, milk, clarified butter and some forms of beans. On the contrary, foods containing high levels of fat, caffeine or alcohol should be avoided. This is much the same advice as conventionally given in the West.

Poor sleep quality may contribute to the effects of chronic fatigue syndrome and Ayurvedic principles recommend the consumption of warm milk with a small quantity of added honey. There is some definite scientific truth behind such advice as milk is major provider of tryptophan, a dietary component which helps in the formation of the sleep-promoting hormone, seratonin.

Homeopathy

While therapeutic approaches such as homeopathy have received bad press as of late, there are many people who believe that this kind of treatment can have a beneficial effect on chronic fatigue syndrome. It is highly unlikely that a conventional medical doctor will suggest or even agree with any homeopathic treatment, but nevertheless you may find it useful.

The general idea behind homeopathy is the concept of treating like with like. That is to say that a disease can be treated with compounds which normally induce symptoms similar to those caused by the illness itself. The belief is that symptoms of illness are the body's reaction to the disease process, and as such the stimulation of these symptoms is believed to assist the body in ridding itself of disease.

Homeopathy preparations are made by diluting the purported active substance in water until little remains. Such dilution is believed to leave a lasting effect on the water itself. There are a number of homeopathic substances used in the treatment of chronic fatigue syndrome and the exact kind will depend on the results of a full homeopathic examination, a holistic approach which considers your whole life in the context of illness rather than just the physical symptoms.

One treatment used is **gelsemium**, which is particularly warranted in cases of muscle weakness and drowsiness. More commonly, however, **kali phosphoricum** is used in chronic fatigue syndrome as it is indicated in cases of muscle weakness as well as insomnia, anxiety and depression. As with other approaches, improvements in diet and exercise are also considered useful.

Chronic fatigue syndrome is often considered as having occurred as a result of exposure to the Epstein-Barr virus which causes glandular fever, also know as mononucleosis. Homeopaths consider a compound known as **mercurius solubilis** to be of use when cases of chronic fatigue involve swollen lymph nodes and sore throats.

It is important that, whatever approach you decide to take, you inform your conventional medical practitioner to ensure that any medicines you are taking do not interact with any holistic therapies you have.

Osteopathy

Osteopathy considers that all diseases are a result of the improper alignment and positioning of the body's muscles and bones. It has been established that osteopathy is highly effective for muscle aches and pains, particularly in the case of lower back problems. The case for its use in chronic fatigue syndrome is less well established, but it may be of some use in symptomatic improvement.

In terms of osteopathy, chronic fatigue syndrome is caused by a prolonged stress response within the body. The effect of this is that the lymphatic system, which drains toxins and fluids from different compartments of the body, becomes altered. The hyperactivity of the nervous system due to stress causes the lymphatic vessels to become faulty, such that toxins are allowed to accumulate within the body. In particular, this is considered to be the root cause of the muscular pain, loss of mental clarity and poor memory associated with chronic fatigue syndrome.

Spinal manipulation and gentle massage of the head allows the proper drainage of toxins into the blood. The liver can then process the toxins so that they are able to be excreted.

It is expected that symptoms will worsen upon such treatment, owing to the release of the trapped toxic compounds, but over time symptomatic relief is considered to occur.

The osteopathic treatment protocol as a whole involves a **massage routine, a gentle series of exercises and dietary advice**. Yet again, diet is implicated in the causes of chronic fatigue syndrome, and that is why this book placed such emphasis on dietary advice as an adjunct to conventional and holistic therapies.

Electromagnetic Stress

The increasing array of gadgets and electrical technologies with which we are surrounded in modern life may have an untoward effect on our bodies. It has been well established that electromagnetism is a phenomenon that is detected and used by animals such as birds for navigation. It has also been purported that the natural electromagnetism of the Earth itself may have an effect on things like blood pressure. Some believe that it also can have an effect on conditions such as chronic fatigue syndrome.

Glandular cells are particularly sensitive to the effect of radiation, and this includes electromagnetic radiation and natural atmospheric radiation. This theory links in with the adrenal fatigue theory behind the true cause of chronic fatigue syndrome. There is not yet a medically established link between these phenomena but some forms of magnetic treatments and electromagnetic frequency generators have been purported to help in the relief of symptoms of chronic fatigue syndrome.

Geopathic Stress

Similar to the effects of electromagnetic radiation, natural radiation emitted by the Earth beneath us has been proposed as a cause for some forms of chronic fatigue syndrome. Some parts of the Earth are considered to be more harmful than others, depending on the levels of background radiation released. This is particularly the case in the presence of granite, which is naturally radioactive though at a very low level.

Unfortunately, research by scientists in the West is lacking and as such this is generally a phenomenon confined to other parts of the world. A practitioner of such methods might employ the use of certain instruments to determine the effects of such phenomena on the body. As of the present moment, this approach remains untested by the scientific method and it is not necessarily recommended.

The Buteyko Method

Named after a Ukrainian doctor of the same name, this is an approach that considers the nature of your breathing and the effects it has on the health of the body. It was initially used to treat asthma, and may be worth considering in terms of overcoming breathing-related responses to stressful stimuli.

Much like the breathing advocated by yoga, the Buteyko method is most likely to have a psychological effect on your management of your symptoms as a result of learning how to physically control part of your response to your symptoms and their causes. It is particularly useful in overcoming hyperventilation. As with any holistic method, the Buteyko method should be discussed with your physician as an adjunct to medical therapies and may not be enough on its own to fully combat your condition.

The Lightning Process

The Lightning Process is an approach which places great significance on the influence of the adrenal system and sympathetic nervous system on stress response. The idea is that the body and brain have responded in a certain way to an initial infection or other stimulus, and have become stuck in this mode of operation.

Initially, the stressor is considered to be something such as the Epstein-Barr virus or some kind of chemical toxin. When recovery does not occur as it should following the conclusion of the disease process, the illness is prolonged. When this prolongation is combined with the fear of never fully recovering it can leave the body in a mode of constant stress response.

As part of this stress response the body produces hormones such as adrenaline, noradrenaline and cortisol which over time cause exhaustion, alterations in blood sugar and immune system suppression. This in turn stresses the body and creates a positive feedback loop. The cumulative effect of this influence on the body is manifested in chronic fatigue syndrome.

There is only anecdotal evidence of the efficacy of the Lightning Process, rather than concrete scientific evidence, and the cost of attending the relevant course may be prohibitive. That said, there are some aspects of treatment according to this plan that coincide with the kinds of proven benefits that can be obtained from cognitive behavioural therapy.

The major difference is that the Lightning Process claims that the stress loop is broken by the stimulation of new neurological pathways due to the adoption of different movements, postures and the asking of questions relevant to resolution of your condition. Once again, it must be said that such treatments should be discussed with your physician before they are used as an adjunct to conventional therapies.

Cookbook

This chapter aims to further crystallise the dietary information in previous chapters in order to give you a better understanding of the kind of diet that you could adopt to improve the symptoms of chronic fatigue syndrome. This approach will be exemplified by a choice of recipes to enable you to make the first steps towards your recovery.

Grains form a large part of the average modern Western diet, but refined carbohydrates are well known for their effect on energy levels. The consumption of simple sugars, found in processed cakes and desserts in particular, leads to an initial energy burst but soon causes feelings of fatigue as a result of the after-effects of a spike in insulin.

As such, any diet formulated to combat chronic fatigue syndrome should restrict intake of sources of refined carbohydrates such as white bread and pasta. These can be substituted for whole grain products which cause a slower release of energy, allowing it to last longer. Additionally, the consumption of certain carbohydrates may contribute to the production of serotonin which, as mentioned earlier, contributes to better sleep. However, if you find yourself lethargic after consumption of such products then they should be avoided.

In fact, some sufferers of chronic fatigue syndrome have thrived on a low carbohydrate intake, instead choosing fruits and vegetables as the mainstay of their diet. Furthermore, any grains they did choose to eat were gluten-free. As mentioned in an earlier chapter, this may aid you if there is an irritable bowel component to your condition. Examples of such grains are oatmeal, barley, quinoa and brown rice.

Artificial sweeteners such as aspartame are generally not recommended as a replacement product for the simple sugars that you ought to eliminate from your diet. Avoiding aspartame may improve your body's perception of pain and also may positively influence your cognitive function.

Another additive to avoid is monosodium glutamate, commonly marked on food product packaging as MSG. It is a flavour enhancer which has been implicated in causing hypersensitivity reactions. Such reactions involve the immune system and may contribute towards the overall stress exerted on your body and exacerbating the symptoms of chronic fatigue syndrome.

Having several good protein sources is vital to ensure that muscle health is maintained and therefore muscle fatigue and weakness is reduced as much as possible. It is important to consume healthy sources of protein such as cold water fish and lean meats and poultry to ensure that you get access to a wide range of different amino acids. That said, fried forms of these foods, as are common on the high street, ought to be avoided due to the high fat and salt content. A good alternative protein source to animal products is to be found in the many varieties of beans and other legumes.

While often given a bad rap, and falling in and out of favour with mass media, fats are actually essential for the proper functioning of the body. Our cell membranes are composed of different kinds of fats and our nervous system cannot work without them. It is true, however, that not all fats are born equal. Some kinds of fats are more beneficial than others, and omega-3 and omega-6 fats are particularly important when consumed in the correct ratio. These fats are responsible for many things, but you'll feel the benefit of their inclusion in your diet through their effects of easing joint pain and improving blood flow.

One of the best sources of these kinds of fats is cold water, oily fish, but you can also find a substantial amount in different nuts and seeds. In particular, flaxseed is known for its useful fat content and it can be conveniently used in muesli and granola recipes for breakfast. Additionally, extra virgin olive oil should be incorporated into your diet as an extremely valuable source of omega-3.

Dairy products are significant source of nutrients and calories in some parts of the world, particularly India and Europe. However, in many people dairy products are not processed particularly well and can contribute to a feeling of lethargy and tiredness. Many sufferers of chronic fatigue syndrome have reported improvement in their symptoms following limitation of non-fermented dairy products such as milk. It may be best to stick to fermented products such as yogurt which promote the growth of beneficial bacteria in your gut, and subsequently improve metabolism and overall health and well-being. Again, this may have a positive influence on the digestive side of your condition.

As mentioned previously, it is important to avoid becoming overly reliant on stimulants such as coffee. Though the initial energy burst may be helpful, the so-called comedown after this short period may prove to be detrimental. This is not to mention the fact that the initial energy burst may exacerbate feelings of anxiety and may promote a general over-excitability which may not be useful in the long run. There are many substitutes which can be consumed instead of coffee though they do not provide the same kind of buzz. These include a "coffee" made of dandelion roots and chamomile tea, which is world renowned for its calming effects on the nervous system.

As chronic fatigue syndrome ultimately affects the way in which energy is generated in your cells, it is important to follow the advice of the dietary chapter of this book which explains the need to increase your intake of certain vitamins and minerals in order to boost your metabolism and this energy levels.

An additional way in which you can improve your energy levels is to consume foods which contain a high level of antioxidants, such as blueberries. Many patients with chronic fatigue syndrome have elevated levels of methemoglobin in their blood, which indicates that their body is under oxidative stress. Antioxidant-rich foods are essential in combating this by their binding to the oxidation get substances and the subsequent exertion of them by the body.

Blueberries in particular are useful for this function as they have the additional properties of having a protective effect on nerve cells and red blood cells. Overall, this ought to help improve symptoms of fatigue.

While chronic fatigue syndrome seems to have many causative and contributory factors, this book has extolled some of the ways in which you can increase energy levels by either directly influencing these factors or through other means. With the belief that our diets make up a large part of who we are, this book will be concluded with a selection of recipes which you can use to get started on your road to recovery.

Recipes

Breakfast

Rice Porridge

3 oz rice flakes or ground rice

15 oz rice milk

A few drops of Vanilla essence

1/2 tsp cinnamon

Salt to taste

1 tsp honey

1 tsp flaxseed

Blueberries

1) Cook the rice flakes in the rice milk in a saucepan over a medium heat for 15 minutes, stirring frequently.

2) Add the cinnamon, salt and honey and mix well.

3) Add the flaxseed and a handful of blueberries.

4) Serve hot.

Layered Greek Yogurt with Nuts and Berries

1 cup organic Greek yogurt

1/2 cup blueberries

1 tbsp flaxseed

2 tbsp almonds, chopped

1/2 cup strawberries, sliced

Honey for drizzling

1) Pour half of the yogurt into a suitable container or bowl.

2) Layer the blueberries, almonds and flax on top.

3) Cover with the rest of the yogurt.

4) Garnish with a few almonds and a drizzle of honey.

Flour-free Mini Banana Pancakes

1 ripe banana, mashed

2 eggs

Coconut oil

2 tbsp flax seeds

Pinch of vanilla

Pinch of cinnamon

Pinch of pumpkin pie spice

1) Mash the banana with a fork.

2) Whisk the eggs in a bowl, then add the banana, flax seeds, vanilla, cinnamon and pumpkin pie spice, and mix well.

3) Heat the coconut oil in a pan.

4) Add enough of the banana batter to form a circle of 2 inches in diameter.

5) When the pancake begins to bubble in the center, flip it over.

6) Serve immediately with berries and organic maple syrup if desired.

Lunch

Edamame and Almond Salad

1 lb edamame beans, shelled

1 tbsp sesame seed oil

1 tbsp rice wine vinegar

2 tbsp soy sauce

1 tsp chilli sauce

1/4 cup sliced almonds, toasted

2 spring onions, chopped

1/4 cup fresh basil, chopped

1/4 cup fresh mint, chopped

1) Cook the edamame beans in boiling water until soft. Drain and let cool.

2) Mix the remaining ingredients in a bowl.

3) Add the edamame beans to the dressing and mix.

Red Pepper, Sweet Potato and Tomato Soup

3 red peppers, deseeded and chopped

2 medium onions, peeled and chopped

2 celery stalks, chopped

14 oz can of tomatoes

2-3 sweet potatoes, peeled and chopped

Chicken or vegetable stock (preferably low sodium and organic)

1 clove of garlic, chopped

Olive oil

Salt and black pepper to taste

1) Chop and sauté the red peppers and onions in olive oil for a few minutes.

2) Add the celery, garlic and sweet potato, and sauté for a few minutes.

3) Add the tomatoes and cover the vegetables in stock. Season with salt and pepper to taste.

4) Cook until all the vegetables are soft. Blend the soup, ensuring that some chunks remain.

Chicken and Avocado Ranch Salad

2 cups romaine lettuce, chopped

1/2 cup carrots, shredded

1/2 cup red bell pepper, sliced

3 oz chicken breast, grilled and sliced

1/4 avocado, mashed

1 1/2 tbsp organic Ranch dressing

1) Add the romaine lettuce, carrots, bell pepper and chicken to a bowl.

2) Mash the avocado with the Ranch dressing.

3) Add the dressing to the salad, toss and serve.

Dinner

Fish Cakes

1/2 lb smoked mackerel or canned tuna

2 -3 medium sweet potatoes, peeled and chopped

1 onion, chopped

1 fennel bulb, chopped finely

1 egg, lightly beaten

Lemon juice

Gluten-free breadcrumbs

Olive oil

1) Cook the sweet potatoes in salted boiling water until soft.

2) Sauté the onion and fennel until softened.

3) Drain and mash the sweet potato roughly.

4) Flake the fish and add it to the sweet potato mash.

5) Add the onion and fennel to the sweet potato mash.

6) Mix the contents of the mash together and add an egg to bind it all.

7) Form the mash into fish cakes and leave them to cool in the refrigerator.

8) Gluten-free breadcrumbs can be used to coat the fish cakes.

9) The fish cakes can be fried or grilled and served with a side salad.

Pumpkin Soup

1 tbsp olive oil

1 medium butternut squash, peeled and chopped

1 medium onion, peeled and chopped

2 stalks celery, chopped

2 cloves garlic, crushed

6 cups organic chicken or vegetable stock

1 large orange, juiced

Live natural yoghurt to garnish

Pinch of salt and black pepper

1) Heat the oil in a large saucepan and cook the pumpkin, onion, celery and garlic for 5 minutes at a medium heat.

2) Add the stock to the saucepan and cover. Cook for a further 25-30 minutes.

3) Blend the contents of the saucepan until of a smooth consistency.

4) Return to the saucepan and season with salt, pepper and orange juice.

5) Can be served hot or cold with a generous tablespoon of fresh yoghurt swirled in.

Crockpot Beef Stew

2 lbs organic beef, chopped

2 tbsp olive oil

1 cup celery, diced

3 cloves of garlic, peeled and minced

1 medium onion, peeled and diced

1 sprig of fresh thyme

1 sprig of fresh rosemary

1 tbsp Worcestershire sauce

1 cup carrots, chopped

1 can of tomatoes, chopped

1 tsp salt

1/2 tsp black pepper

3 sweet potatoes, peeled and chopped

1/2 cup beef broth

1) Put all ingredients into a crockpot and cook for 4 to 8 hours.

Snacks

Avocado Fries

1 avocado, sliced into thick wedges

1 egg, whisked

1/2 cup unsweetened coconut flakes

1/4 cup coconut flour

1/2 tsp chilli powder

1/4 tsp ground cumin

1/2 tsp salt

Coconut oil

1) Sprinkle the avocado wedges with half of the salt.

2) Mix the remainder of the salt with the cumin, chilli powder and coconut flakes until finely chopped.

3) Coat each avocado wedge in egg, then coconut flour. Re-coat in egg and then in the coconut flakes.

4) Fry each wedge on each side for a maximum of 1 minute per side so that they are browned.

Eggs Mimosa

6 hard-boiled eggs, peeled

2 avocados, halved

1 clove of garlic, crushed

1 tbsp olive oil

Pinch of salt and black pepper

10 lettuce leaves

1) Reserve 1 egg, and halve the remainder.

2) Put the yolks in a mixing bowl. Blend them with the avocado, salt, pepper and olive oil.

3) Spoon this mixture back into the egg halves.

4) Sieve the remaining egg whites and sprinkle on top of the prepared eggs.

5) Repeat step 4 with the remaining egg yolks.

6) Place each half egg on a lettuce leaf to serve.

Green Smoothie

2 cups spinach

1/2 avocado

Handful of strawberries

Handful of blueberries

1) Blend all ingredients together. **Best consumed immediately**.

Conclusion

Thank you for reading this full book. I have written all the information about 'Chronic Fatigue Syndrome'. Don't be frustrated about Chronic Fatigue. Knowledge can go a long way in treatment and prevention.